Mediterranean Guidebook

A Step-By-Step Guide To Everything You Need To Get Started With The Mediterranean Diet. The Solution For Lifelong Health And Amazing Meals

Written By

HOLLIE MCCARTHY, RDN

Table of Contents

INTRODUCTION

Thank you for purchasing this book!

Many studies associate **the Mediterranean diet with a reduced risk of cardiovascular diseases.** Positive effects derive from a set of characteristics of this diet. Among the many:

- **low content of saturated fats**
- **the abundance of unsaturated fats, such as omega-3 from fish and dried fruit and the oleic acid from extra virgin olive oil**
- **the reduced consumption of salt in favor of spices and aromas**.

All elements contribute to keep **under control the values of cholesterol and triglycerides,** for the benefit of heart health, and **to prevent diseases such as hypertension**. For the same reasons, the Mediterranean diet also proves to be **an ally against metabolic syndrome, i.e. that set of conditions (obesity, diabetes, hypertension, dyslipidemia) that exposure to high cardiovascular risk**.

Enjoy your reading!

BREAKFAST

Johnnycakes (Vegan)

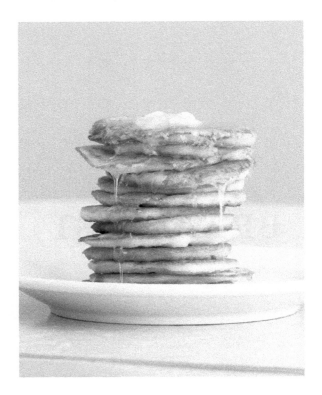

SERVES: 4

INGREDIENTS

- 1 cup yellow cornmeal
- 1 teaspoon salt
- 1 teaspoon sugar
- 1½ cups boiling water, plus more if needed
- Canola or grapeseed oil, for frying

DIRECTIONS

1. In a medium bowl, combine the cornmeal, salt, and sugar and mix well. Slowly stir in the water, mixing until smooth. Add up to 3 tablespoons of additional water if the mixture is too thick. Preheat the oven to 225°F.

2. On a griddle or large skillet, heat a thin layer of oil over medium heat, adding enough oil to coat. Drop large tablespoonfuls of the batter onto the hot griddle and cook until small bubbles appear on the top, about 5 minutes. Be careful not to burn. Flip the Johnnycakes and cook until the second side is browned, another 4 to 5 minutes.

3. Transfer cooked Johnnycakes to a heatproof platter and keep warm in the oven while cooking the rest.

Maple-Pecan Waffles (Vegan)

SERVES: 4

INGREDIENTS

- 1¾ cups all-purpose flour
- ⅓ cup coarsely ground pecans
- 1 tablespoon baking powder
- ½ teaspoon salt
- 1½ cups soy milk
- tablespoons pure maple syrup
- tablespoons vegan margarine, melted

DIRECTIONS

1. Lightly oil the waffle iron and preheat it. Preheat the oven to 225°F.
2. In a large bowl, combine the flour, pecans, baking powder, and salt. Set aside.
3. In a medium bowl, whisk together the soy milk, maple syrup, and margarine. Add the wet ingredients to the dry ingredients and blend with a few swift strokes, mixing until just combined.
4. Ladle ½ to 1 cup of the batter (depending on the instructions with your waffle iron) onto the hot
5. waffle iron. Cook until done, 3 to 5 minutes for most waffle irons. Transfer the cooked waffles to a heatproof platter and keep warm in the oven while cooking the rest of the waffles.

Pumpkin Waffles With Cranberry Syrup (Vegan)

SERVES: 4

INGREDIENTS

- ½ cup whole berry cranberry sauce
- ⅓ cup cranberry juice
- 2 tablespoons pure maple syrup
- 1 tablespoon vegan margarine
- 1¾ cups all-purpose flour
- 1 tablespoon baking powder
- ½ teaspoon salt
- 1 teaspoon ground cinnamon
- ½ teaspoon ground ginger
- ½ teaspoon ground allspice
- ¼ teaspoon ground nutmeg
- 1 cup soy milk
- ½ cup canned solid-pack pumpkin
- 2 tablespoons canola or grapeseed oil
- 1 teaspoon pure vanilla extract

DIRECTIONS

1. In a small saucepan, heat the cranberries, cranberry juice, maple syrup, and margarine over medium heat. Cook, stirring, until hot and well blended, about 5 minutes. Keep warm over very low heat until ready to serve.

2. Lightly oil the waffle iron and preheat it. Preheat the oven to 225°F. In a large bowl, combine the flour, sugar, baking powder, salt, cinnamon, ginger, allspice, and nutmeg. Set aside.

3. In a separate large bowl, whisk together the soy milk, pumpkin, oil, and vanilla until well blended. Add the liquid ingredients to the dry ingredients and blend with a few swift strokes until just combined.

4. Ladle ½ cup to 1 cup of the batter (depending on the instructions with your particular waffle iron)

5. onto the hot waffle iron. Cook until done, 3 to 5 minutes for most waffle irons. Transfer cooked waffles to a heatproof platter and keep warm in the oven while making the rest of the waffles.

Lemon-Kissed Blueberry Waffles (Vegan)

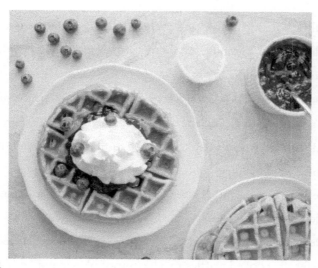

SERVES: 4

INGREDIENTS

- 1½ cups all-purpose flour
- ½ cup old-fashioned oats
- ¼ cup sugar
- teaspoons baking powder
- ½ teaspoon salt
- 1 teaspoon ground cinnamon
- 2 cups soy milk
- 1 tablespoon fresh lemon juice
- 1 teaspoon lemon zest
- ¼ cup vegan margarine, melted
- ½ cup fresh blueberries

DIRECTIONS

1. Lightly oil the waffle iron and preheat it. Preheat the oven to 225°F.

2. In a large bowl, combine the flour, oats, sugar, baking powder, salt, and cinnamon. Set aside.

3. In a separate large bowl, whisk together the soy milk, lemon juice, lemon zest, and margarine. Add the wet ingredients to the dry ingredients and blend with a few swift strokes, mixing until just combined. Fold in the blueberries.

4. Ladle ½ to 1 cup of the batter (depending on the instructions with your waffle iron) onto the hot

5. waffle iron. Cook until done, 3 to 5 minutes for most waffle irons.

6. Transfer the cooked waffles to a heatproof platter and keep warm in the oven while cooking the rest.

LUNCH

Thai peanut shrimp curry

SERVES: 2

INGREDIENTS

- 2 tbsp. Green Curry Paste
- 1 cup Vegetable Stock
- 1 cup Coconut Milk
- 6 oz. Precooked Shrimp
- 5 oz. Broccoli Florets
- 3 tbsp. Cilantro, chopped
- 2 tbsp. Coconut Oil
- 1 tbsp. Peanut Butter
- 1 tbsp. Soy Sauce (or coconut)
- Juice of 1/2 Lime
- 1 medium Spring Onion, chopped
- 1 tsp. Crushed Roasted Garlic
- 1 tsp. Minced Ginger
- 1 tsp. Fish Sauce
- 1/2 tsp. Turmeric
- 1/4 tsp. Xanthan Gum
- 1/2 cup Sour Cream (for topping)

DIRECTIONS

1. Start by adding 2 tbsp. coconut oil in a pan over medium heat.
2. When the coconut oil is melted and the pan is hot, add the 1 tsp. Roasted garlic, 1 tsp. minced ginger, and 1 spring onion (chopped). Allow to cook for about a minute, and then add 1 tbsp. green curry paste, and 1/2 tsp. turmeric.

3. Add 1 tbsp. soy sauce (or Coconut Aminos), 1 tsp. fish sauce, and 1 tbsp. peanut butter to the pan and mix together well.

4. Add 1 cup of vegetable stock and 1 cup of coconut milk (from the carton). Stir well and then add another 1 tbsp. green curry paste.

5. Let simmer for a few minutes. In the meantime, measure out 6 oz. pre-cooked shrimp.

6. Add 1/4 tsp. xanthan gum to the curry and mix well.

7. Once your curry begins thickening up a little bit, add the broccoli florets and stir well.

8. Chop 3 tbsp. fresh cilantro and add to the pan.

9. Finally, once you are happy with the consistency of the curry, add the shrimp and lime juice from 1/2 lime, and mix everything.

10. Let simmer for a few minutes. Taste and season with salt and pepper if needed.

11. Serve! You can stir in 1/4 cup of sour cream per serving.

NUTRITIONAL VALUES

455 Calories, 35g Fats, 9g Net Carbs, and 27g Protein.

Grilled cheese sandwich

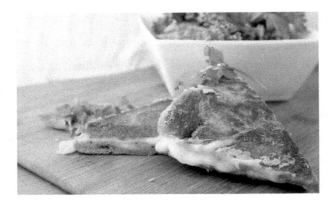

SERVES: 1

INGREDIENTS

Bun Ingredients

- 2 large Eggs
- 2 tbsp. Almond Flour
- 1 1/2 tbsp. Psyllium Husk Powder
- 1/2 tsp. Baking Powder
- 2 tbsp. Soft Butter

Fillings & Extras

- 2 oz. Cheddar Cheese (or white cheddar, if you're feeling frisky)
- 1 tbsp. Butter, for frying

DIRECTIONS

1. Let 2 tbsp. butter come to room temperature in a mug. Once it's soft, add 2tbsp. Almond Flour, 1 1/2 tbsp. Psyllium Husk, and 1/2 tsp. Baking Powder.

2. Mix this as well as you can so that a thick dough is formed.

3. Add 2 large eggs and continue mixing. You want a pretty thick dough. If your dough isn't thick, continue mixing the dough – it will thicken up as you mix it (this can take up to 60 seconds).

4. Pour the dough into a square container or bowl. Level it off and clean off the sides that it comes out as level as you can get it.

5. Microwave for about 90-100 seconds. You will have to check the doneness of it to make sure it doesn't need longer.

6. Remove from the container or bowl by flipping it upside down and lightly tapping the bottom. Cut it in half using a bread knife.

7. Measure out the cheese you can and stick it between the buns.

8. Bring 1 tbsp. butter to heat in a pan over medium heat. Once hot, add a bun and allow cooking in the butter. This should be absorbed by the bread as you cook and give a delicious, crisp outside.

9. Serve up with a side salad for some delicious grilled cheese!

NUTRITIONAL VALUES

793 Calories, 70g Fats, 7g Net Carbs, and 29g Protein.

DINNER

Creamy butter shrimp

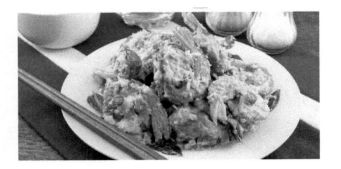

SERVES: 3

INGREDIENTS

- 1/2 oz. Parmigiano Reggiano, grated
- 2 tbsp. Almond Flour
- 1/2 tsp. Baking Powder
- 1/4 tsp. Curry Powder
- 1 tbsp. Water
- 1 large Egg
- medium Shrimp
- 3 tbsp. Coconut Oil

Creamy Butter Sauce

- 2 tbsp. Unsalted Butter
- 1/2 small Onion, diced
- 1 clove Garlic, finely chopped
- 2 small Thai Chilies, sliced

Garnish

- 2 tbsp. Curry Leaves
- 1/2 cup Heavy Cream
- 1/3 oz. Mature Cheddar
- Salt and Pepper to Taste
- 1/8 tsp. Sesame Seeds

DIRECTIONS

1. Remove the shells of the shrimps but leave the tail part if you'd like

2. Pat the cleaned shrimps dry with paper towels.

3. In a bowl, add 0.5 oz. grated Parmigiano Reggiano, 2 tbsp. almond flour, 1/2 tsp. baking powder and 1/4 tsp. curry powder (optional). Mix well. Gently cut the surface of the shrimps and devein. Clean well Into the mixture, add in 1 egg and 1 tbsp. water. Mix well until smooth.

4. Preheat a pan on medium heat. Add in 3 tbsp. coconut oil. Once the oil is hot, generously coat the shrimps with the batter and pan-fry the shrimps. Do these two to three at a time.

5. Wait until the shrimps turn golden brown and then remove them from the pan. Put on a cooling rack. Pan-fry extra batter if any left.

6. Preheat a pan to medium-low heat. Add in 2 tbsp. unsalted butter. Once the butter has melted, add in 1/2 chopped onion.

7. Wait until the onion turns translucent and then add in finely chopped garlic, sliced Thai chilies, and 2 tbsp. Curry leaves. Stir-fry everything until fragrant.

8. Add in the battered shrimp and coat well with the sauce.

9   Garnish with sesame seeds and serve! Goes well with cauliflower fried rice.

10   This makes a total of 3 servings.

NUTRITIONAL VALUES

570 Calories, 52g Fats, 3g Net Carbs, and 14g Protein.

Buffalo chicken jalapeno popper casserole

SERVES: 6

INGREDIENTS

- 6 small Chicken Thighs
- 6 slices Bacon
- 3 medium Jalapenos (De-seed if you aren't a fan of spicy)
- oz. Cream Cheese
- 1/4 cup Mayonnaise
- 4 oz. Shredded Cheddar
- 2 oz. Shredded Mozzarella Cheese
- 1/4 cup Frank's Red Hot
- Salt and Pepper to Taste

DIRECTIONS

1   De-bone all chicken thighs and pre-heat oven to 400F. Season chicken thighs well with salt and pepper then lay on a cooling rack over a cookie sheet wrapped in foil. Bake chicken thighs for 40 minutes at 400F.

2   Once your timer hits 20 minutes, start on the filling. Chop 6 slices of bacon into pieces and put into a pan over medium heat.

3   Once the bacon is mostly crisped, add jalapenos into the pan.

4   Once jalapenos are soft and cooked, add cream cheese, mayo, and frank's red hot to the pan. Mix and season to taste.

5   Remove chicken from the oven and let cool slightly. Once they are cool enough, remove the skins from the chicken.

6   Lay chicken into a casserole dish, then spread cream cheese mixture over it, then top with cheddar and mozzarella cheese.

7   Bake for 10-15 minutes at 400F. Broil for 3-5 minutes to finish. Optional: Top with extra jalapenos before you broil.

8   Let cool for 5 minutes. Slice and serve up!

SNACKS

Pecan butter chia seed blondies

SERVES: 5

INGREDIENTS

- 2 1/4 cups Pecans, roasted
- 1/2 cup Chia Seeds
- 1/4 cup butter, melted
- 1/4 cup Erythritol, powdered
- 3 tbsp. SF Torani Salted Caramel
- drops Liquid Stevia
- 3 large Eggs
- 1 tsp. Baking Powder
- 3 tbsp. Heavy Cream
- 1 pinch Salt

DIRECTIONS

1. Preheat oven to 350F. Measure out 2 1/4 cup pecans and bake for about 10 minutes. Once you can smell a nutty aroma, remove nuts
2. Grind 1/2 cup whole chia seeds in a spice grinder until a meal forms.
3. Remove chia meal and place in a bowl. Next, grind 1/4 cup Erythritol in a spice grinder until powdered. Set in the same bowl as the chia meal.
4. Place 2/3 of roasted pecans in the food processor.
5. Process nuts, scraping sides down as needed until the smooth nut butter is formed.

6. Add 3 large eggs, 10 drops of liquid stevia, 3 tbsp. SF Salted Caramel Torani Syrup, and a pinch of salt to the chia mixture. Mix this well.

7. Add pecan butter to the batter and mix again.

8. Using a rolling pin, smash the rest of the roasted pecans into chunks inside of a plastic bag.

9. Add crushed pecans and 1/4 cup melted butter into the batter.

10. Mix batter well and then adds 3 tbsp. Heavy cream and 1 tsp. Baking Powder. Mix everything well.

11. Measure out the batter into a 9×9 tray and smooth out.

12. Bake for 20 minutes or until desired consistency.

13. Let cool for about 10 minutes. Slice off the edges of the brownie to create a uniform square. This is what I call "the bakers treat" – yep, you guessed it!

14. Snack on those bad boys while you get them ready to serve to everyone else. The so-called "best part" of the brownie is the edges, and that's why you deserve to have all of it.

15. Serve up and eat to your heart's (or rather macros) content!

This makes 16 total Pecan Butter Chia Seed Blondies

NUTRITIONAL VALUES

174 Calories, 11g Fats, 1g Net Carbs, and 9g Protein.

Cilantro infused avocado lime sorbet

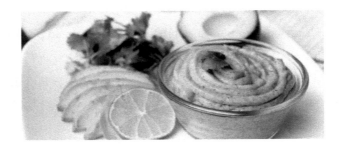

SERVES: 4

INGREDIENTS

- 2 medium Hass Avocados
- 1/4 cup NOW Erythritol, Powdered
- 2 medium Limes, Juiced & Zested
- 1 cup Coconut Milk
- 1/4 tsp. Liquid Stevia
- 1/4 – 1/2 cup Cilantro, Chopped

DIRECTIONS

1. Slice avocados in half. Use the butt of a knife and drive it into the pits of the avocados. Slowly twist and pull the knife until put is removed.
2. Slice avocado half vertically through the flesh, making about 5 slices per half of an avocado. Use a spoon to carefully scoop out the pieces. Rest pieces on foil and squeeze the juice of 1/2 lime over the tops.
3. Store avocado in the freezer for at least 3 hours. Only start the next step 2 1/2 hours after you put the avocado in the freezer.

4. Using a spice grinder, powder 1/4 cup NOW Erythritol until a confectioner's sugar type of consistency is achieved.

5. In a pan, bring 1 cup Coconut Milk (from Carton) to a boil.

6. Zest the 2 limes you have while coconut milk is heating up.

7. Once the coconut milk is boiling, add lime zest and continue to let the milk reduce in volume.

8. Once you see that the coconut milk is starting to thicken, remove it and place it into a container. It should have reduced by about 25%.

9. Store the coconut milk mixture in the freezer and let it completely cool.

10. Chop 1/4 – 1/2 cup cilantro, depending on how much cilantro flavor you'd like.

11. Remove avocados from the freezer. They should be completely frozen along with the lime juice. The lime juice should have helped them not turn brown.

12. Add avocado, cilantro, and juice from 1 1/2 lime into the food processor. Pulse until a chunky consistency is achieved.

13. Pour coconut milk mixture over the avocados in the food processor. Add 1/4 tsp. Liquid Stevia to this.

14. Pulse mixture together until desired consistency is reached. This takes about 2-3 minutes.

15. Return to freezer to freeze, or serve immediately!

NUTRITIONAL VALUES

180 Calories, 16g Fats, 5g Net Carbs, and 2g Protein.

SIDE DISHES

Easy, delicious coleslaw

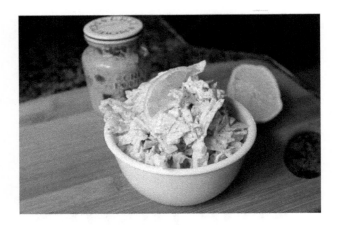

SERVES: 1

INGREDIENTS

- 1/4 Head Savoy Cabbage
- 1/3 cup Mayonnaise
- 1 Tbsp. Lemon Juice
- 1 tsp. Dijon Mustard
- 1/4 tsp. Garlic Powder
- 1/4 tsp. Onion Powder
- 1/4 tsp. Pepper
- 1/8 tsp. Paprika
- Pinch Salt

DIRECTIONS

1 Chop the 1/4 Head Savoy Cabbage lengthwise so that each of the strands come off of the cabbage clean.

2 Mix the 1/3 Cup Mayonnaise, 1 Tbsp. Lemon Juice, 1 tsp. Dijon

3 Mustard, 1/4 tsp of Garlic Powder, Onion Powder, Black Pepper, and 1/8 tsp. of Paprika. You can also add a pinch of salt if you'd like.

4 3 Measure out servings and serve!

Cheesy thyme waffles

SERVES: 1

INGREDIENTS

- 1/2 Head Cauliflower, Riced
- 1 Cup Finely Shredded
- Mozzarella Cheese
- 1 Cup Collard Greens, Packed
- 1/3 Cup Parmesan Cheese
- 2 Large Eggs
- 2 Stalks Green Onion
- 1 Tbsp. Sesame Seed
- 1 Tbsp. Olive Oil
- 2 tsp. Fresh Chopped Thyme
- 1 tsp. Garlic Powder
- 1/2 tsp. Ground Black Pepper
- 1/2 tsp. Salt

DIRECTIONS

1. Prep your cauliflower, spring onion, and thyme by cutting the cauliflower into florets, slicing the spring onion into small slices, and ripping the thyme off of the stems.
2. In a food processor, rice the cauliflower by pulsing it until a crumbly texture is formed.
3. Add the spring onion, thyme, and collard greens to the mixture and continue pulsing until everything is well combined.

4 Scoop the mixture out into a large mixing bowl.

5 Add the 1 Cup Mozzarella Cheese, 1/3 cup Parmesan Cheese, 2 Large

6 Eggs, 1 Tbsp. Sesame Seed, 1 Tbsp. Olive Oil, 1 tsp. Garlic Powder, 1/2 tsp. Black Pepper, and 1/2 tsp. Salt.

7 Mix everything well until a loose batter is formed.

8 Heat your waffle iron until it's ready to go, then spoon mixture onto the waffle iron evenly.

DESSERT

Vegan Tiramisù

SERVES: 6

INGREDIENTS

- 1 cup firm tofu, drained and pressed dry
- 1 (8-ounce) container vegan cream cheese
- ½ cup vegan vanilla ice cream, softened
- 1 teaspoon pure vanilla extract
- ⅓ cup plus 1 tablespoon superfine sugar
- ½ cup coffee, cooled to room temperature
- 2 tablespoons coffee liqueur
- 1 vegan pound cake, homemade (see Vegan Pound Cake) or store-bought, or other white or yellow cake, cut into ½-inch-thick slices
- 1 tablespoon unsweetened cocoa powder

DIRECTIONS

1. In a food processor, combine the tofu, cream cheese, ice cream, vanilla, and ⅓ cup of the sugar. Process until smooth and well blended.
2. In a small bowl, combine the coffee, the remaining 1 tablespoon sugar, and the coffee liqueur.

3. Arrange a single layer of cake slices in an 8-inch square baking pan and brush with half of the coffee mixture. Sprinkle with half of the cocoa. Spread half the tofu mixture over the cake. Arrange another layer of cake slices on top of the tofu mixture. Brush with the remaining coffee mixture and spread evenly with the remaining tofu mixture. Sprinkle with the remaining cocoa. Chill 1 hour before serving.

Indian Pudding

SERVES: 6

INGREDIENTS

- 3½ cups plain or vanilla soy milk
- ½ cup sugar
- ½ cup dark molasses
- ½ cup yellow cornmeal
- ½ teaspoon salt
- ½ teaspoon ground allspice
- ½ teaspoon ground cinnamon
- ¼ teaspoon ground ginger

DIRECTIONS

1. Preheat the oven to 350°F. Grease a 2-quart gratin dish or 9-inch square baking pan and set aside.
2. In a large saucepan, combine the soy milk, sugar, and molasses over medium heat and cook, stirring, until blended.
3. Slowly add the cornmeal, whisking to incorporate. Cook, stirring until thickened, 5 to 7 minutes. Stir in the salt, allspice, cinnamon, and ginger and remove from the heat.
4. Pour the mixture into the prepared pan. Bake until the center is set, about 1 hour.

Sweet Vermicelli Pudding

SERVES: 6

INGREDIENTS

- 2 tablespoons vegan margarine
- 8 ounces sevian noodles, vermicelli noodles, or angel hair pasta
- ½ cup unsalted shelled pistachio nuts
- 2 cups plain or vanilla soy milk
- 1 cup unsweetened coconut milk
- ¼ cup sugar
- ¼ cup golden raisins
- ½ teaspoon ground cardamom
- 1½ teaspoons rosewater or pure vanilla extract

DIRECTIONS

1. In a large skillet, heat the margarine over medium heat. Break the noodles into 2-inch pieces and add them to the skillet along with ¼ cup each of the almonds and pistachios. Cook, stirring until the noodles turn golden. Do not brown.
2. Stir in the soy milk and coconut milk and bring to simmer. Add the sugar, raisins, and cardamom and simmer for 10 minutes.
3. Stir in the rosewater, then transfer to a serving dish and sprinkle with the remaining almonds and pistachios. Serve warm or at room temperature.

Chocolate And Walnut Farfalle

SERVES: 4

INGREDIENTS

- ½ cup chopped toasted walnuts
- ¼ cup vegan semisweet chocolate pieces
- ounces farfalle
- 2 tablespoons vegan margarine
- ¼ cup sugar

DIRECTIONS

1   In a food processor or blender, grind the walnuts and chocolate pieces until crumbly. Do not overprocess. Set aside.

2   In a pot of boiling salted water, cook the farfalle, stirring occasionally, until al dente, about 8 minutes. Drain well and return to the pot.

3   Add the margarine and sugar and toss to combine and melt the margarine.

4   Transfer the noodle mixture to a serving bowl. Add the nut and chocolate mixture and toss to combine. Serve warm.

Fresh Cherry-Vanilla Bread Pudding

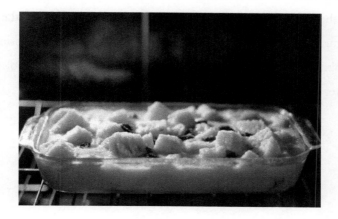

SERVES: 6

INGREDIENTS

- 2 cups cubed white bread
- 2 cups pitted and halved cherries
- 2 cups plain or vanilla soy milk
- ounces soft silken tofu, drained
- ⅔ cup sugar
- 2 teaspoons pure vanilla extract
- ½ cup flaked sweetened coconut

DIRECTIONS

1   Preheat the oven to 350°F. Grease a 9-inch square baking pan. Spread the bread cubes in the prepared baking pan. Sprinkle evenly with the cherries and set aside.

2   In a blender or food processor, combine the soy milk, tofu, sugar, and vanilla and blend until smooth.

3   Pour the liquid mixture over the bread and cherries, pressing the bread to saturate with the liquid. Sprinkle the coconut on top, pressing into the mixture. Bake until firm, about 45 minutes. Allow to cool for 15 minutes and serve. Or refrigerate, 2 hours, to serve chilled.

Chocolate Bread Pudding with Rum Sauce

SERVES: 6

INGREDIENTS

- ⅓ cup unsweetened cocoa powder
- ¼ cup applesauce
- 2 cups plain or vanilla soy milk
- ⅔ cup sugar
- ½ teaspoon ground cinnamon
- Pinch salt
- 2 teaspoons pure vanilla extract
- 2 cups white bread, torn into small pieces
- ½ cup semisweet vegan chocolate chips
- ½ cup vegan margarine, softened
- ½ cup confectioners' sugar
- 2½ tablespoons dark rum

DIRECTIONS

1   Preheat the oven to 350°F. Grease an 8-inch springform pan and set it aside. In a large bowl, combine the cocoa and applesauce, stirring to blend. Stir in the soy milk, sugar, cinnamon, salt, and 1 teaspoon of vanilla. Mix in the bread and chocolate chips.

2   Scrape the mixture into the prepared pan, pressing with your hands to spread evenly. Bake until set, about 45 minutes. Remove from the oven and set aside to cool on a wire rack.

3   In a large bowl, combine the margarine and sugar and beat with an electric mixer at high speed until incorporated for about 2 minutes. Add the rum and remaining 1 teaspoon of vanilla and beat on high speed for 3 minutes.

4   Remove the sides of the springform pan, cut the pudding into wedges and transfer to dessert plates. Spoon the sauce over the pudding and serve.

260 - Granola-Stuffed Baked Apples

SERVES: 6

INGREDIENTS

- ½ cup vegan granola, homemade (see Granola) or store-bought
- 2 tablespoons creamy peanut butter or almond butter
- 1 tablespoon vegan margarine
- 1 tablespoon pure maple syrup
- ½ teaspoon ground cinnamon
- Granny Smith or other firm baking apples
- 1 cup apple juice

DIRECTIONS

1   Preheat the oven to 350°F. Grease a 9 x 13-inch baking pan and set it aside. In a medium bowl, combine the granola, peanut butter, margarine, maple syrup, and cinnamon and mix well.

2   Core the apples and stuff the granola mixture into the centers of the apples, packing tightly.

3   Place the apples upright in the prepared pan. Pour the apple juice over the apples and bake until tender, about 1 hour. Serve warm.

Pecan And Date-Stuffed Roasted Pears

SERVES: 4

INGREDIENTS

- firm-ripe pears, cored
- 1 tablespoon fresh lemon juice
- ½ cup finely chopped pecans
- dates, pitted and chopped
- 1 tablespoon vegan margarine
- 1 tablespoon pure maple syrup
- ¼ teaspoon ground cinnamon
- ⅛ teaspoon ground ginger
- ½ cup pear, white grape, or apple juice

DIRECTIONS

1   Preheat the oven to 350°F. Grease a shallow baking dish and set it aside. Halve the pears lengthwise and use a melon baller to scoop out the cores. Rub the exposed part of the pears with lemon juice to avoid discoloration.

2   In a medium bowl, combine the pecans, dates, margarine, maple syrup, cinnamon, and ginger and mix well.

3   Stuff the mixture into the centers of the pear halves and arrange them in the prepared baking pan. Pour the juice over the pears. Bake until tender, 30 to 40 minutes. Serve warm.

Banana Fritters with Caramel Sauce

SERVES: 6

INGREDIENTS

- ripe bananas, mashed
- 2 tablespoons pure maple syrup
- 2 tablespoons sugar
- ⅓ cup plain or vanilla soy milk
- ⅔ cup all-purpose flour
- ½ teaspoon ground cinnamon
- ¼ teaspoon salt
- 2 teaspoons baking powder
- 1 tablespoon vegan margarine, melted
- Canola or other neutral oil, for frying
- Caramel Sauce, homemade or store-bought

DIRECTIONS

1   In a large bowl, combine the bananas, maple syrup, sugar, and soy milk. Stir in the flour, cinnamon, salt, and baking powder, then mix in the margarine until well blended.

2   In a large skillet, heat a thin layer of oil over medium-high heat. When the oil is hot, carefully place spoonfuls of the banana mixture into the skillet. Do not crowd. Fry until golden brown on one side, then turn and fry the other side, about 6 to 8 minutes total. Drain the cooked fritters on paper towels.

3   Arrange the fritters on dessert plates and drizzle with caramel sauce. Serve warm.

MEDITERRANEAN SEAFOOD

Crab Stuffed Avocado

SERVES: 4

INGREDIENTS

- 1 pound cooked, chilled, rinsed, and picked over fresh crabmeat
- 1 cup mayonnaise
- 1 teaspoon lemon pepper seasoning
- 1 cup chopped celery
- 1/4 cup sweet pickle relish
- 1/2 cup chopped scallions
- 2/3 cup sliced almonds
- or 3 avocados

DIRECTIONS

1   Place the crabmeat in a paper towel–lined bowl. Allow standing for 15 minutes. Remove paper towel.

2   Mix mayonnaise, lemon pepper, celery, pickle relish, and almonds together. Gently toss with crabmeat.

3   Slice avocado in 2 around the seed. Split and remove seed and discard.

4   Fill seed hole and tops of avocado with crab mixture.

5   Serve immediately.

Crab Stuffed Mushrooms

SERVES: 4

INGREDIENTS

- 1 pound large mushrooms
- tablespoons butter
- tablespoons finely chopped onion
- 1 (3 ounces) package cream cheese, softened
- tablespoons prepared Dijon–style mustard
- 1/2 ounces crabmeat
- 1/4 cup chopped water chestnuts
- tablespoons chopped pimento peppers
- tablespoons grated Parmesan cheese

DIRECTIONS

1   Preheat oven to 400F.

2   Remove stems from the mushrooms, retaining the caps.

3   Chop the stems.

4   In a medium saucepan, melt the butter. Brush the mushroom caps with melted butter. In the remaining butter, cook and stir the chopped mushroom stems and onions until tender.

5   Gradually mix the cream cheese and mustard into the saucepan. Continue stirring until smooth.

6   Stir in the crabmeat, water chestnuts, and pimentos. Heat until warm. Stuff the mushroom caps with the crabmeat mixture.

7   Sprinkle the stuffed caps with Parmesan cheese.

8   In a shallow pan, bake the caps at 400F for 10 to 15 minutes or until hot.

Crabby Potatoes

SERVES: 4

INGREDIENTS

- large potatoes, baked or microwaved
- until tender, then cooled
- 1 pound lump crabmeat
- 1/2 cup chopped green bell pepper
- 1/2 cup chopped onion
- tablespoons mayonnaise
- teaspoons dry mustard
- 1 tablespoon prepared brown mustard
- 1 teaspoon paprika
- tablespoons seafood seasoning
- 1/2 cup butter, melted

DIRECTIONS

1   Preheat oven to 350 degrees F.
2   Cut potatoes in half lengthwise; scoop out pulp, leaving the shell intact. Set pulp aside.
3   In a large bowl, mix crabmeat, green pepper, onion, mayonnaise, mustards, paprika, and 1 tablespoon seafood seasoning.
4   Place potato skins on a cookie sheet. Spoon crab mixture into each potato half.
5   Top with potato pulp.

6   Sprinkle remaining seafood seasoning over potato halves.

7   Bake 5 to 10 minutes, until heated through but not dried. Remove from
    oven; pour melted butter over.

Crabmeat Imperial

SERVES: 2

INGREDIENTS

- 1 pound lump crabmeat, picked over to remove any shell 1/2 cup scallions, finely chopped
- 1/2 cup green bell pepper, finely chopped
- 1/4 cup chopped pimentos
- 1 egg yolk
- 1 teaspoon dry mustard
- artichoke hearts, coarsely chopped
- tablespoons paprika
- 1 cup mayonnaise
- 1/4 cup freshly grated Parmesan cheese
- 1/4 cup seasoned bread crumbs
- Salt and black pepper

DIRECTIONS

1 Preheat oven to 375F.
2 In a large bowl, combine the crabmeat, scallions, bell pepper, pimento, egg yolk, dry mustard, artichoke hearts, paprika, and one–half cup of mayonnaise.
3 Stir until well–mixed and season with salt and pepper to taste.
4 Spoon the crabmeat mixture into four one–cup baking dishes; then cover with the remaining mayonnaise.

63

5   Sprinkle Parmesan and bread crumbs on top and bake in the hot oven for 15 to 20 minutes until heated through.

6   Serve immediately.

Pecan–Crusted Crab Cakes with Sweet Pepper Sauce

SERVES: 4

INGREDIENTS

- 1/3 cup pecan halves
- 1 slice firm-textured white bread, torn
- 2 tablespoons mayonnaise
- 2 teaspoons lemon juice
- 1 teaspoon Dijon mustard
- 1 egg yolk
- 4 ounces (1/4 pound) lump crab meat
- 1 tablespoon minced chives
- 1 1/2 tablespoons butter
- Sweet Pepper Sauce
- 1 large red bell pepper (1/2 pound, coarsely chopped
- 1 tablespoon olive oil
- 1 tablespoon plus 1 teaspoon balsamic vinegar
- Salt and cayenne, to taste

DIRECTIONS

1   Place pecans and torn bread in a blender or small food processor. Pulse until pecans are finely chopped and bread is crumbly.

2   In a medium bowl combine mayonnaise, lemon juice, mustard, and egg yolk; blend well. Add crab and chives; stir gently to mix, breaking up large lumps. Stir in 6 tablespoons of pecan−bread crumbs.

3   Place remaining crumbs on a plate. Form crab mixture into 4 cakes, about 2 inches in diameter.

4   Dredge crab cakes in crumbs, pressing gently to help the mixture adhere.

5   In a medium skillet (nonstick one), melt butter over medium−low heat. Add crab cakes, cover the pan and sauté, turning over once, about 5 minutes total, until they are hot in the center and nicely browned on both sides.

6   To serve, spoon pepper sauce onto 2 salad plates. Place 2 crab cakes on each plate. Garnish with whole chives and lemon wedges

Cream Puffs with Crab Filling

SERVES: 6 to 8

INGREDIENTS

Cream Puffs

- 1 cup water
- 1/2 cup butter
- 1 cup flour
- 1/4 teaspoon salt
- 4 eggs

Crab Filling

- 11 ounces cream cheese (8 ounces and 3 ounces)
- 1 cup mayonnaise or sour cream
- 1 teaspoon lemon juice
- 1/4 teaspoon horseradish
- 2 tablespoons finely chopped onion
- 7 ounces fresh crab or shrimp

DIRECTIONS

1. Mix crab filling a day ahead and refrigerate.
2. Heat water, butter, and salt to a rolling boil.
3. Reduce heat and quickly stir in flour with a wooden spoon until the mixture leaves the sides of the pan in a ball.
4. Remove from heat and add eggs, 1 at a time, beating after each addition until mixture is smooth and not glossy.

5   Drop 1 tablespoon (size is optional) on a baking sheet. Bake at 400 degrees F for approximately 25 minutes until golden brown.

6   Let puffs completely cool before slicing.

French Fried Jimmy Crabs

SERVES: 4

INGREDIENTS

- 1 dozen medium−size male crabs(washed and scrubbed in water with legs, back shells, and innards removed)
- 1 pound backfin crab meat
- 1 scant cup flour
- 1 scant cup milk
- 1 teaspoon salt
- 1 teaspoon celery seed
- teaspoon parsley
- 1 egg
- 1 teaspoon Old Bay seasoning
- 1 tablespoon vegetable oil
- Enough vegetable oil for deep frying

DIRECTIONS

1 Combine all ingredients except crab, crab meat, and vegetable oil to make a batter.
2 Stir one tablespoon of vegetable oil into the batter.
3 Fill crab crevices where innards were removed with crab meat and press the crab meat firmly into the crevice to secure.

4   Holding each stuffed crab with tongs, dip into the batter. Then place into the deep fryer filled with very hot vegetable oil.

5   Completely cover the crab and fry individually for seven minutes or until golden.

Maryland Crab Cakes

SERVES: 6

INGREDIENTS

- slices white bread
- 3/4 cup olive oil
- eggs, separated
- 1/4 teaspoon dry mustard
- 1/2 teaspoon salt
- teaspoon Worcestershire sauce
- 1 1/2 pounds crabmeat
- Paprika
- tablespoons butter

DIRECTIONS

1 Trim crusts from bread and lay slices on a shallow platter. Pour oil over them and let stand until bread is thoroughly saturated. Use forks to break into small pieces.

2 Combine egg yolks with mustard, salt, and Worcestershire sauce. Beat lightly. Stir in bread and crab meat.

3 Gently fold in stiffly beaten egg whites, and shape mixture into patties. Sprinkle with paprika and sauté in heated butter until golden on both sides.

Maryland Fried Softshell Crabs

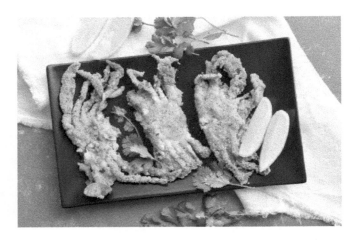

SERVES: 6

INGREDIENTS

- soft-shell crabs
- 1 1/2 cups milk
- 1/2 teaspoon pepper
- teaspoons salt
- 1/2 cup flour
- Shortening (for frying)
- Tartar sauce

DIRECTIONS

1   Wash cleaned soft shell crabs.

2   Dry well. Soak in milk seasoned with salt and pepper for 15 minutes; roll in flour.

3   Heat shortening and fry crabs until crisp and brown.

4   Drain on absorbent paper.

5   Serve with tartar sauce or on sandwich bread.

Salt and Pepper Soft-shell crab

SERVES: 4

INGREDIENTS

- 2 soft-shell crabs, cleaned and cut into 8 pieces
- 2 birds eye chili - chopped
- 2 garlic cloves - crushed
- 1 spring onion - finely chopped
- ½ beaten egg
- 40g potato flour
- ½ teaspoon salt
- ⅖ teaspoon sugar
- A pinch of teaspoon five-spice powder
- A pinch of teaspoon ginger powder
- Vegetable oil for cooking
- Whole leaves of an Iceberg lettuce

DIRECTIONS

1   Wash and dry the crabs. Lay the soft shell crabs on a board and cut into 4 pieces per crab

2   Mix a beaten egg and a little potato flour. Dip crab pieces into the mix then coat well with the remaining potato flour

3   Carefully lower into the hot oil for 2 minutes, turning two or three times, or until golden brown and crisp. Remove from the oil with a slotted spoon and drain on kitchen paper.

4   Meanwhile, add 1 teaspoon of oil to wok, then chili, garlic, spring onions, and stir fry for two seconds return the crab to the wok. Add salt, sugar, five-spice, and ginger powder, and toss all ingredients together for a few seconds.

5   When ready, remove from wok, place onto lettuce leaf garnish, and serve at once.

Crab Enchiladas with Cherry Tomato Salsa

SERVES: 6

INGREDIENTS

- 6 flour tortillas (7 inches in diameter)
- 3 tablespoons corn oil
- 10 ounces fresh lump crabmeat, picked over
- 1 cup grated Jalapeno Jack cheese (about 5 ounces)
- 1 cup shredded fresh spinach leaves
- Cherry Tomato Salsa

DIRECTIONS

Preheat the oven to 300F. Wrap the tortillas tightly in foil and bake for 10 to 15 minutes, until heated through.

In a medium skillet, heat the oil. Add the crabmeat and saute over moderately high heat until heated for 2 to 3 minutes.

Spoon the crabmeat onto the center of the warm tortilla and sprinkle with the cheese and the spinach. Roll the tortillas into cylinders and place on a warmed serving plate, seam-side down. Surround with Cherry Tomato Salsa.

Cherry Tomato Salsa

- 2 pints cherry tomatoes
- 1 large shallot, minced
- 1 large garlic clove, minced
- 2 tablespoons minced fresh coriander
- 1 tablespoon white wine vinegar
- 2 serrano chiles, seeded and minced

- 2 teaspoons fresh lime juice
- 1/4 teaspoon salt

DIRECTIONS

1   In a food processor, coarsely chop the tomatoes, turning the machine on and off. Do not puree.
2   In a medium bowl, combine the chopped tomatoes and their juices with shallot, garlic, coriander, vinegar, chiles, lime juice, and salt.
3   Stir well. Cover with plastic wrap and set aside for at least 2 hours to blend the flavors.

Baked Mahi-Mahi with Dill Sauce

SERVES: 4

INGREDIENTS

- 1/4 cup sour cream
- 1/4 cup plain yogurt
- 1 tablespoon mayonnaise or salad dressing
- 1 tablespoon minced fresh dill or 1 teaspoon dried dill
- 1/2 teaspoon Dijon mustard
- 1/8 teaspoon bottled hot pepper sauce
- Salt & pepper to taste
- Mahi-Mahi Steaks
- 1 tablespoon vegetable oil
- 1 tablespoon lemon juice
- Salt
- White pepper

DIRECTIONS

1   Combine our sour cream, yogurt, mayonnaise, mustard, and hot sauce. Stir in dill; add salt and pepper to taste. Blend well.

2   Allow standing at least 1/2 hour to blend flavors. Serve at room temperature. May be refrigerated for up to 24 hours.

3   Pat fish dry with paper towels. Combine oil and lemon juice; brush on both sides of fish. Season lightly with salt and white pepper.

4   Place an inch apart in a lightly oiled baking dish. Bake at 450F for approximately 15 minutes. When fish tests are done, transfer to warm plates. Spoon Dill Sauce over fish.

Mahi-mahi skewers with seafood butter

SERVES: 4

INGREDIENTS

- bamboo or metal skewers
- ¾cup olive oil
- 1 tablespoon toasted sesame oil Zest and juice of a lemon
- 1 tablespoon chopped fresh parsley
- ¾teaspoon coarse salt
- ¾teaspoon ground black pepper
- pounds skinless mahi-mahi steaks or thick fillets, cut into 1-inch cubes
- 1 lemon, cut into 8 wedges
- cherry or grape tomatoes
- strips bacon, preferably applewood-smoked, cut into 3-inch lengths
- ¾cup Seafood Butter

DIRECTIONS

1   Combine the olive oil, sesame oil, lemon zest, lemon juice, parsley, salt, and black pepper in a 1-gallon zipper-lock bag. Add the mahi-mahi, press out the air, and seal the bag. Refrigerate for up to 12 hours.

2   If you are grilling with bamboo skewers, soak them in water for at least 30 minutes. Light a grill for direct medium heat, about 400¼F. Thread the lemon wedges, tomatoes, and mahi-mahi cubes alternately on the skewers, using about 2 pieces of each per skewer. For the mahi-mahi, wrap each cube on three sides with a piece of bacon, and skewer

3 through the ends of the bacon to secure it. Set aside some of the seafood butter for serving and brush the skewers with the rest.

4 Brush the grill grate and coat with oil. Grill the skewers directly over the heat until the fish looks opaque on the surface, but is still filmy and moist in the center (130¼F on an instant-read thermometer). Drizzle with the reserved sea-food butter and serve with the grilled lemon wedges for squeezing.

Wasabi-drizzled mussels grilled with green tea fumes

SERVES: 4

INGREDIENTS

- Loose green tea leaves, such as bancha or hojicha
- 1 cups Green Tea Ponzu Sauce
- 1 cup tamari or soy sauce
- scallions (green and white parts), finely chopped
- 1 tablespoon grated fresh ginger
- Grated zest and juice of 1 large lemon Grated zest and juice of 1 small lime
- ¾ounce kombu (dried kelp), torn into pieces
- pounds mussels, debearded and scrubbed
- teaspoons wasabi paste

DIRECTIONS

1   Soak the tea leaves in cold water for 30 minutes.

2   Light a grill for direct medium heat, about 350¼F, with smoke. Combine the ponzu sauce, tamari, scallions, ginger, lemon zest and juice, lime zest and juice, and kombu in a disposable aluminum pan large enough to hold the mussels in a single layer (or nearly single). Add the mussels to the pan.

3   Add the soaked tea leaves to the grill as you would wood chips. Put the pan of mussels directly over the heat, close the lid, and cook until the

mussels open, 15 to 20 minutes, spooning the liquid over the mussels a few times.

4   Pluck the mussels from the liquid and transfer them to shallow bowls, discarding any mussels that do not open.

5   Strain the liquid through cheesecloth into another bowl. Pour 1 cup of the strained liquid into a bowl and stir in the wasabi paste. Pour the remaining strained liquid over the mussels. Drizzle with the wasabi mixture and serve.

MEDITERRANEAN PASTA

Spaghetti Caprese

PREP TIME: 8 Minutes

COOKING TIME: 30 Minutes

SERVES 1

INGREDIENTS

- 1 C. fresh tomato, diced
- salt,
- 1 tbsp onion, minced
- 1 pinch pepper
- 1 tbsp olive oil, divided
- 4 oz. spaghetti
- 1/2 tsp sugar
- 1 tbsp fresh basil, chopped

DIRECTIONS

1   Prepare the pasta by following the instructions on the package.
2   Place a large saucepan over medium heat. Heat in it 1/2 tbsp of oil. Sauté in it the onion for 2 min
3   Lower the heat then stir in the tomatoes, sugar, pepper, and salt. Let them cook for 6 min.
4   Stir in the basil with 1/2 tbsp of oil to the sauce. Mix them well. Turn off the heat and let it sit for few minutes.

5   Spoon the sauce over the spaghetti then serve it warm.

6   Enjoy.

NUTRITIONAL VALUES

Calories 587.6, Fat 15.6g, Cholesterol 0.0mg, Sodium 16.6mg, Carbohydrates 95.2g, Protein 16.6g

Pesto Aioli Dressing

PREP TIME: 15 Minutes

COOKING TIME: 15 Minutes

SERVES 20

INGREDIENTS

- 3/4 C. oil
- 1/2 tsp salt
- 1 C. mayonnaise
- 1 clove garlic, minced
- 3/4 C. buttermilk
- hot pepper sauce
- 2 tbsp grated Romano cheese
- 1/4 tsp paprika
- 2 tbsp dried basil

DIRECTIONS

1   Get a small mixing bowl: Mix the mayo with oil.
2   Pour in the buttermilk, cheese, basil, salt, garlic, and hot pepper sauce. Whisk them until they become creamy.
3   Cover the bowl with plastic wrap and let it sit for at least 8 h.
4   Once the time is up, toss the spaghetti with the pesto sauce. Garnish it with some fresh basil.

5   Enjoy.

NUTRITIONAL VALUES

Calories 124.5, Fat 12.3g, Cholesterol 3.9mg, Sodium 157.9mg, Carbohydrates 3.4g, Protein 0.6g

Brenda's Tomato Sauce

PREP TIME: 30 Minutes

COOKING TIME: 60 Minutes

SERVES 6

INGREDIENTS

- 8 large fresh tomatoes, diced
- 1 tsp fresh ground black pepper
- 1/2 C. olive oil
- 1/4 tsp crushed red pepper flakes
- 8 cloves fresh garlic, chopped
- 3/4 C. fresh basil, minced
- 1/2 tsp salt

DIRECTIONS

1 Place a pan over medium heat. Heat in it the oil. Cook in it the garlic for 1 min.
2 Stir in the tomatoes and cook them for 5 min. Add the basil with red pepper, a pinch of salt, and pepper.
3 Let the sauce cook for 6 to 10 min over low heat until it becomes slightly thick.
4 Pour some of the sauce over the spaghetti then serve it warm.
5 Enjoy.

NUTRITIONAL VALUES

Calories 210.8, Fat 18.5g, Cholesterol 0.0mg, Sodium 207.3mg, Carbohydrates 11.2g, Protein 2.5g

Slow cooker Spaghetti

PREP TIME: 10 Minutes

COOKING TIME: 6 Hours

SERVES 6

INGREDIENTS

- 1 lb.. ground beef
- 1 1/2 tsp Italian seasoning
- 2 tbsp instant minced onion
- 4 oz. mushrooms
- 1 tsp salt
- 3 C. tomato juice
- 1/2 tsp garlic powder
- 4 oz. spaghetti, broken into pieces
- 8 oz. tomato sauce

DIRECTIONS

1   Place a crockpot over medium heat. Cook in it the beef for 6 min.
2   Stir in the onion with tomato sauce, mushroom, tomato juice, Italian seasoning, garlic powder and salt.
3   Put on the lid and let them cook for 7 h on low.

4   Once the time is up, add the pasta. Put on the lid and let it cook for 60 min on high.

5   Enjoy.

NUTRITIONAL VALUES

Calories 273.6, Fat 11.8g, Cholesterol 51.4mg, Sodium 966.5mg, Carbohydrates 23.5g, Protein 18.7g

Carbonara Spaghetti

PREP TIME: 5 Minutes

COOKING TIME: 15 Minutes

SERVES 4

INGREDIENTS

- 12 oz. spaghetti
- 3 eggs
- 1 tbsp olive oil
- 1 1/4 C. heavy cream
- 1 onion, chopped
- 2 oz. parmesan cheese
- 4 oz. bacon, diced
- salt and pepper
- 1 clove garlic, chopped

DIRECTIONS

1   Prepare the pasta by following the instructions on the package.
2   Place a pan over medium heat. Heat in it the oil. Cook in it the bacon with onion for 6 min.
3   Add the garlic and cook them for 1 min.
4   Get a mixing bowl: Whisk in it the eggs with cream, a pinch of salt, and pepper.
5   Add them to the onion and bacon mixture. Stir them well and let them cook for 3 to 5 min over low heat.
6   Add the pasta to the sauce and stir it to a coat.

7   Adjust the seasoning of the pasta then serve it warm.

8   Enjoy.

NUTRITIONAL VALUES

Calories 860.4, Fat 52.6g, Cholesterol 273.1mg, Sodium 541.2mg, Carbohydrates 69.7g, Protein 26.4g

Chinese Spaghetti

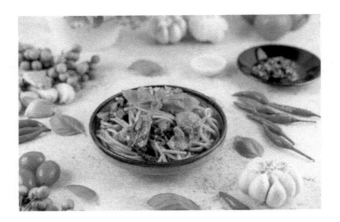

PREP TIME: 20 Minutes

COOKING TIME: 40 Minutes

SERVES 6

INGREDIENTS

- 8 oz. spaghetti, uncooked
- 1 tbsp canola oil
- 1 tbsp cornstarch
- 2 C. fresh snow peas
- 4 tbsp reduced-sodium soy sauce,
- 2 C. carrots, shredded
- divided
- 3 green onions, chopped
- 2 tbsp sesame oil, divided
- 3/8 tsp ground ginger, minced
- 1 lb.. boneless skinless chicken breast,

- 1/2 tsp crushed red pepper flakes
- cut into pieces
- 2 tbsp white vinegar
- 1 tbsp sugar

DIRECTIONS

1   Prepare the pasta by following the instructions on the package.
2   Get a mixing bowl: Mix in it the cornstarch and 1 tbsp soy sauce. Stir in 1 tbsp of sesame oil to make the marinade.
3   Place the chicken in a zip lock bag. Pour over it the sesame oil sauce. Press the bag to seal it and shake it to coat.
4   Place it aside and let it absorb the flavors for 12 min.
5   Get a mixing bowl: Mix in it vinegar, sugar, remaining soy sauce, and sesame oil to make the sauce.
6   Place a large pan over medium heat. Heat in it the canola oil. Add the marinated chicken and cook it for 7 to 10 min until it is done.
7   Drain the chicken and place it aside. Add the carrots with peas then cook them for 6 min.
8   Stir in the green onions, ginger, and pepper flakes. Let them cook for 6 to 7 min until they are done to your liking.
9   Stir in the cooked chicken with vinegar sauce and spaghetti. Cook them for 2 min. Serve your chicken and spaghetti stir fry warm. Enjoy.

NUTRITIONAL VALUES
Calories 337.1, Fat 9.5g, Cholesterol 48.4mg, Sodium 477.5mg, Carbohydrates 38.9g, Protein 22.7g

VEGAN MAIN DISHES

Tempting Tempeh Chili

SERVES: 4

INGREDIENTS

- 1 pound tempeh
- 1 tablespoon olive oil
- 1 medium yellow onion, chopped
- 1 medium green bell pepper, chopped
- 2 garlic cloves, minced
- tablespoons chili powder
- 1 teaspoon dried oregano
- 1 teaspoon ground cumin
- (28-ounce) can crushed tomatoes
- ½ cup water, plus more if needed
- 1½ cups cooked or 1 (15.5-ounce) can pinto beans, drained and rinsed
- 1 (4-ounce) can chop mild green chiles, drained
- Salt and freshly ground black pepper
- 2 tablespoons minced fresh cilantro

DIRECTIONS

1   In a medium saucepan of simmering water, cook the tempeh for 30 minutes. Drain and allow to cool, then finely chop and set aside.

2   In a large saucepan, heat the oil. Add the onion, bell pepper, and garlic, cover, and cook until softened, about 5 minutes. Add the tempeh and cook, uncovered, until golden, about 5 minutes. Add the chili powder, oregano, and cumin. Stir in the tomatoes, water, beans, and chiles. Season with salt and black pepper to taste. Mix well to combine.

3   Bring to a boil, then reduce the heat to low, cover, and simmer for 45 minutes, stirring occasionally, adding a little more water if needed.

4   Sprinkle with cilantro and serve immediately.

Tempeh Cacciatore

SERVES: 4

INGREDIENTS

- 1 pound tempeh, cut thinly sliced
- 2 tablespoons canola or grapeseed oil
- 1 medium red onion, cut into ½-inch dice
- medium red bell pepper, cut into ½-inch dice
- medium carrot, cut into ¼-inch slices
- 2 garlic cloves, minced
- 1 (28-ounce) can diced tomatoes, drained
- ¼ cup dry white wine
- 1 teaspoon dried oregano
- 1 teaspoon dried basil
- Salt and freshly ground black pepper

DIRECTIONS

1   In a medium saucepan of simmering water, cook the tempeh for 30 minutes. Drain and pat dry.

2   In a large skillet, heat 1 tablespoon of the oil over medium heat. Add the tempeh and cook until browned on both sides, 8 to 10 minutes total. Remove from the skillet and set aside.

3   In the same skillet, heat the remaining 1 tablespoon oil over medium heat. Add the onion, bell pepper, carrot, and garlic. Cover, and cook until softened, about 5 minutes.

4   Add the tomatoes, wine, oregano, basil, and salt, and black pepper to taste and bring to a boil. Reduce heat to low, add the reserved tempeh, and simmer, uncovered, until the vegetables are soft and the flavors are well combined for about 30 minutes. Serve immediately.

Indonesian Tempeh In Coconut Gravy

SERVES: 4

INGREDIENTS

- 1 pound tempeh, cut into ¼-inch slices
- 2 tablespoons canola or grapeseed oil
- 1 medium yellow onion, chopped
- 3 garlic cloves, minced
- 1 medium red bell pepper, chopped
- 1 medium green bell pepper, chopped
- 1 or 2 small serrano or other fresh hot chiles, seeded and minced
- 1 (14.5-ounce) can diced tomatoes, drained
- 1 (13.5-ounce) can unsweetened coconut milk
- Salt and freshly ground black pepper
- ½ cup unsalted roasted peanuts, ground or crushed, for garnish
- 2 tablespoons minced fresh cilantro, for garnish

DIRECTIONS

1   In a medium saucepan of simmering water, cook the tempeh for 30 minutes. Drain and pat dry.

2   In a large skillet, heat 1 tablespoon of the oil over medium heat.

3   Add the tempeh and cook until golden brown on both sides, about 10 minutes. Remove from the skillet and set aside.

4   In the same skillet, heat the remaining 1 tablespoon oil over medium heat. Add the onion, garlic, red and green bell peppers, and chiles.

5   Cover and cook until softened, about 5 minutes. Stir in tomatoes and coconut milk. Reduce heat to low, add the reserved tempeh, season with salt and pepper to taste, and simmer, uncovered, until the sauce is slightly reduced about 30 minutes. Sprinkle with peanuts and cilantro and serve immediately.

Ginger-Peanut Tempeh

SERVES: 4

INGREDIENTS

- 1 pound tempeh, cut into ½-inch dice
- 2 tablespoons canola or grapeseed oil
- medium red bell pepper, cut into ½-inch dice
- 3 garlic clove, minced
- small bunch green onions, chopped
- 2 tablespoon grated fresh ginger
- 2 tablespoons soy sauce
- 1 tablespoon sugar
- ¼ teaspoon crushed red pepper
- 1 tablespoon cornstarch
- 1 cup water
- 1 cup crushed unsalted roasted peanuts
- 2 tablespoons minced fresh cilantro

DIRECTIONS

1   In a medium saucepan of simmering water, cook the tempeh for 30 minutes. Drain and pat dry. In a large skillet or wok, heat the oil over medium heat.

2   Add the tempeh and cook until lightly browned about 8 minutes.

3   Add the bell pepper and stir-fry until softened, about 5 minutes. Add the garlic, green onions, and ginger and stir-fry until fragrant, 1 minute.

4   In a small bowl, combine the soy sauce, sugar, crushed red pepper, cornstarch, and water. Mix well, then pour into the skillet. Cook, stirring, for 5 minutes, until slightly thickened. Stir in the peanuts and cilantro. Serve immediately.

Tempeh with Potatoes And Cabbage

SERVES: 4

INGREDIENTS

- 1 pound tempeh, cut into ½-inch dice
- 2 tablespoons canola or grapeseed oil
- 1 medium yellow onion, chopped
- 1 medium carrot, chopped
- 1½ tablespoons sweet Hungarian paprika
- 2 medium russet potatoes, peeled and cut into ½-inch dice
- 3 cups shredded cabbage
- 1 (14.5-ounce) can diced tomatoes, drained
- ¼ cup dry white wine
- 1 cup vegetable broth, homemade (see Light Vegetable Broth) or store-bought Salt and freshly ground black pepper
- ½ cup vegan sour cream, homemade (see Tofu Sour Cream) or store-bought (optional)

DIRECTIONS

1   In a medium saucepan of simmering water, cook the tempeh for 30 minutes. Drain and pat dry.

2   In a large skillet, heat 1 tablespoon of the oil over medium heat. Add the tempeh and cook until golden brown on both sides, about 10 minutes. Remove tempeh and set aside.

3   In the same skillet, heat the remaining 1 tablespoon oil over medium heat.

4   Add the onion and carrot, cover, and cook until softened, about 10 minutes. Stir in the paprika, potatoes, cabbage, tomatoes, wine, and broth and bring to a boil. Season with salt and pepper to taste.

5   Reduce the heat to medium, add the tempeh, and simmer, uncovered, for 30 minutes, or until the vegetables are tender and the flavors are blended. Whisk in the sour cream, if using, and serve immediately.

Southern Succotash Stew

SERVES: 4

INGREDIENTS

- 10 ounces tempeh
- 2 tablespoons olive oil
- 1 large sweet yellow onion, finely chopped
- 2 medium russet potatoes, peeled and cut into ½-inch dice
- 1 (14.5-ounce) can diced tomatoes, drained
- 1 (16-ounce) package frozen succotash
- 2 cups vegetable broth, homemade (see Light Vegetable Broth) or store-bought, or water
- 2 tablespoons soy sauce
- 1 teaspoon dry mustard
- 1 teaspoon sugar
- ½ teaspoon dried thyme
- ½ teaspoon ground allspice
- ¼ teaspoon ground cayenne
- Salt and freshly ground black pepper

DIRECTIONS

1   In a medium saucepan of simmering water, cook the tempeh for 30 minutes. Drain, pat dry, and cut into 1-inch dice.

2   In a large skillet, heat 1 tablespoon of the oil over medium heat. Add the tempeh and cook until browned on both sides, about 10 minutes. Set aside.

3   In a large saucepan, heat the remaining 1 tablespoon oil over medium heat. Add the onion and cook until softened, 5 minutes.

4   Add the potatoes, carrots, tomatoes, succotash, broth, soy sauce, mustard, sugar, thyme, allspice, and cayenne. Season with salt and pepper to taste.

5   Bring to a boil, then reduce heat to low and add the tempeh. Simmer, covered, until the vegetables are tender, stirring occasionally, about 45 minutes.

6   About 10 minutes before the stew is finished cooking, stir in the liquid smoke. Taste, adjust seasonings if necessary

7   Serve immediately.

Baked Jambalaya Casserole

SERVES: 4

INGREDIENTS

- 10 ounces tempeh
- 2 tablespoons olive oil
- 1 medium yellow onion, chopped
- 1 medium green bell pepper, chopped
- 2 garlic cloves, minced
- 1 (28-ounce) can diced tomatoes, undrained
- ½ cup white rice
- 1½ cups vegetable broth, homemade (see Light Vegetable Broth) or store-bought, or water
- 1½ cups cooked or 1 (15.5-ounce) can dark red kidney beans, drained and rinsed
- 1 tablespoon chopped fresh parsley
- 1½ teaspoons Cajun seasoning
- 1 teaspoon dried thyme
- ½ teaspoon salt
- ¼ teaspoon freshly ground black pepper

DIRECTIONS

1   In a medium saucepan of simmering water, cook the tempeh for 30 minutes. Drain and pat dry. Cut into ½-inch dice. Preheat the oven to 350°F.

2   In a large skillet, heat 1 tablespoon of the oil over medium heat. Add the tempeh and cook until browned on both sides, about 8 minutes. Transfer the tempeh to a 9 x 13-inch baking dish and set it aside.

3   In the same skillet, heat the remaining 1 tablespoon oil over medium heat. Add the onion, bell pepper, and garlic. Cover and cook until the vegetables are softened, about 7 minutes.

4   Add the vegetable mixture to the baking dish with the tempeh. Stir in the tomatoes with their liquid, the rice, broth, kidney beans, parsley, Cajun seasoning, thyme, salt, and black pepper. Mix well, then cover tightly and bake until the rice is tender about 1 hour. Serve immediately.

Tempeh and Sweet Potato Shepherd's Pie

SERVES: 4

INGREDIENTS

- 8 ounces tempeh
- 3 medium sweet potatoes, peeled and cut into ½-inch dice
- 2 tablespoons vegan margarine
- ¼ cup plain unsweetened soy milk
- Salt and freshly ground black pepper
- 2 tablespoons olive oil
- 1 medium yellow onion, finely chopped
- 2 medium carrots, chopped
- 1 cup frozen peas, thawed
- 1 cup frozen corn kernels, thawed
- 1½ cups Mushroom Sauce
- ½ teaspoon dried thyme

DIRECTIONS

1   In a medium saucepan of simmering water, cook the tempeh for 30 minutes. Drain and pat dry. Finely chop the tempeh and set it aside.

2   Steam the sweet potatoes until tender, about 20 minutes. Preheat the oven to 350°F. Mash the sweet potatoes with margarine, soy milk, and salt and pepper to taste. Set aside.

3   In a large skillet, heat 1 tablespoon of the oil over medium heat. Add the onion and carrots, cover, and cook until soft, about 10 minutes. Transfer to a 10-inch baking pan.

4   In the same skillet, heat the remaining 1 tablespoon oil over medium heat. Add the tempeh and cook until browned on both sides, 8 to 10 minutes. Add the tempeh to the baking pan with the onion and carrots. Stir in the peas, corn, and mushroom sauce. Add the thyme and salt and pepper to taste. Stir to combine.

5   Spread the mashed sweet potatoes on top, using a spatula to spread evenly to the edges of the pan. Bake until the potatoes are lightly browned and the filling is hot, about 40 minutes. Serve immediately.

Basic Simmered Seitan

SERVES: 4

INGREDIENTS

Seitan

- 1¾ cups wheat gluten flour (vital wheat gluten)
- ½ teaspoon salt
- ½ teaspoon onion powder
- ¼ teaspoon sweet paprika
- 1 tablespoon olive oil
- 2 tablespoons soy sauce
- 1⅔ cups cold water

Simmering Liquid:

- 2 quarts water
- ½ cup soy sauce
- 2 garlic cloves, crushed

DIRECTIONS

1   Make the seitan: In a food processor, combine the wheat gluten flour, nutritional yeast, salt, onion powder, and paprika. Pulse to blend.

2   Add the oil, soy sauce, and water and process for a minute to form a dough. Turn the mixture out onto a lightly floured work surface and knead until smooth and elastic, about 2 minutes.

3   Make the simmering liquid: In a large saucepan, combine the water, soy sauce, and garlic.

4   Divide the seitan dough into 4 equal pieces and place in the simmering liquid. Bring just to a boil over medium-high heat, then reduce heat to medium-low, cover, and simmer gently, turning occasionally, for 1 hour. Turn off the heat and allow the seitan to cool in the liquid. Once cool, the seitan can be used in recipes or refrigerated in the liquid in a tightly sealed container for up to a week or frozen for up to 3 months.

Stuffed Baked Seitan Roast

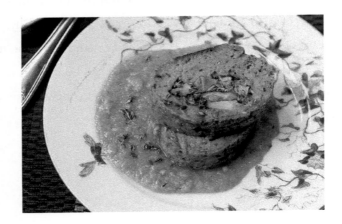

SERVES: 6

INGREDIENTS

- 1 recipe Basic Simmered Seitan, uncooked
- 1 tablespoon olive oil
- 1 small yellow onion, minced
- 1 celery rib, minced
- ½ teaspoon dried thyme
- ½ teaspoon dried sage
- ½ cup water, or more if needed
- Salt and freshly ground black pepper
- 2 cups fresh bread cubes
- ¼ cup minced fresh parsley

DIRECTIONS

1   Place the raw seitan on a lightly floured work surface and stretch it out with lightly floured hands until it is flat and about ½ inch thick.

2   Place the flattened seitan between two sheets of plastic wrap or parchment paper. Use a rolling pin to flatten it as much as you can (it will be elastic and resistant). Top with a baking sheet weighed down with a gallon of water or canned goods and let it rest while you make the stuffing.

3   In a large skillet, heat the oil over medium heat. Add the onion and celery. Cover and cook until soft, 10 minutes. Stir in the thyme, sage, water, and salt and pepper to taste.

4   Remove from heat and set aside. Place the bread and parsley in a large mixing bowl. Add the onion mixture and blend well, adding a little more water if the stuffing is too dry. Taste, adjusting seasonings if necessary. if necessary. Set aside.

5   Preheat the oven to 350°F. Lightly oil a 9 x 13-inch baking pan and set it aside. Roll out the flattened seitan with a rolling pin until it is about ¼ inch thick. Spread the stuffing across the surface of the seitan and roll it up carefully and evenly. Place the roast seam side down in the prepared baking pan. Rub a little oil on the top and sides of the roast and bake, covered for 45 minutes, then uncover and bake until firm and glossy brown, about 15 minutes longer.

6   Remove from the oven and set aside for 10 minutes before slicing. Use a serrated knife to cut it into ½-inch slices. Note: For the easiest slicing, make the roast ahead and cool completely before slicing. Slice all or part of the roast and then reheat in the oven, tightly covered, for 15 to 20 minutes, before serving.

Seitan Pot Roast

SERVES: 4

INGREDIENTS

- 1 recipe Basic Simmered Seitan
- 2 tablespoons olive oil
- 3 to 4 medium shallots, halved lengthwise
- 1 pound Yukon Gold potatoes, peeled and cut into 2-inch chunks
- ½ teaspoon dried savory
- ¼ teaspoon ground sage
- Salt and freshly ground black pepper
- Horseradish, to serve

DIRECTIONS

1   Follow the directions for making Basic Simmered Seitan, but divide the seitan dough into 2 pieces instead of 4 before simmering. After the seitan has cooled in its broth for 30 minutes, remove it from the saucepan and set it aside.

2   Reserve the cooking liquid, discarding any solids.

3   Reserve 1 piece of the seitan (about 1 pound) for future use by placing it in a bowl and covering it with some of the reserved cooking liquid.

4   Cover and refrigerate until needed. If not using within 3 days, cool the seitan completely, wrap tightly, and freeze.

5   In a large saucepan, heat 1 tablespoon of the oil over medium heat. Add the shallots and carrots. Cover and cook for 5 minutes.

6   Add the potatoes, thyme, savory, sage, and salt and pepper to taste. Add 1½ cups of the reserved cooking liquid and bring to a boil.

7   Reduce heat to low and cook, covered, for 20 minutes.

8   Rub the reserved seitan with the remaining 1 tablespoon oil and the paprika. Place the seitan on top of the simmering vegetables.

9   Cover and continue cooking until the vegetables are tender, about 20 minutes more.

10   Cut the seitan into thin slices and arrange on a large serving platter surrounded by the cooked vegetables. Serve immediately, with horseradish on the side.

COOKING CONVERSION CHART

TEMPERATURE	
FAHRENHEIT	CELSIUS
100 °F	37 °C
150 °F	65 °C
200 °F	93 °C
250 °F	121 °C
300 °F	150 °C
325 °F	160 °C
350 °F	180 °C
375 °F	190 °C
400 °F	200 °C
425 °F	220 °C
450 °F	230 °C
500 °F	260 °C
525 °F	270 °C
550 °F	288 °C

WEIGHT	
IMPERIAL	METRIC
1/2 oz	15 g
1 oz	29 g
2 oz	57 g
3 oz	85 g
4 oz	113 g
5 oz	141 g
6 oz	170 g
8 oz	227 g
10 oz	283 g
12 oz	340 g
13 oz	369 g
14 oz	397 g
15 oz	425 g
1 lb	453 g

MEASUREMENT			
CUP	**ONCES**	**MILLILITERS**	**TABLESPOON**
1/16 cup	1/2 oz	15 ml	1
1/8 cup	1 oz	30 ml	3
1/4 cup	2 oz	59 ml	4
1/3 cup	2.5 oz	79 ml	5.5
3/8 cup	3 oz	90 ml	6
1/2 cup	4 oz	118 ml	8
2/3 cup	5 oz	158 ml	11
3/4 cup	6 oz	177 ml	12
1 cup	8 oz	240 ml	16
2 cup	16 oz	480 ml	32
4 cup	32 oz	960 ml	64
5 cup	40 oz	1180 ml	80
6 cup	48 oz	1420 ml	96
8 cup	64 oz	1895 ml	128

Lightning Source UK Ltd.
Milton Keynes UK
UKHW020635100621
385271UK00011B/751